The
Diet Secret

A Step by Step Guide for Sustainable Fat
Loss

Keegan Brown

ISBN: 1542622247
ISBN-13: 9781542622240

To my entire family and to my friends, who are always supportive in everything I do.

To my mom, dad, sister, brother, and grandparents for always pushing me to be the best version of myself. Without them, this book wouldn't have been written.

CONTENTS

ACKNOWLEDGMENTS

There are way too many people for me to thank who have helped me in one way or another to write this book. I would like to thank Sheila Juenger and the Maple Woods Community Fitness Center staff for allowing me to follow my passion. Thank you to my papa Larry for always telling me to do the things that make me happy. You have shaped my life in too many ways for me to list and for which I'm very grateful. Thank you also to my grandma Sandy for always being loving, caring, and supportive; to my grandma Julie for pushing me always to be a better person and for being supportive; to my brother and sister for putting up with me but always being supportive; to my friend Brandon for helping me value hard work; to my friend Ethan Dillon for always pushing me to do better in and out of the gym; to my friend Tony Powers for helping me when I first got into personal training; to my friend Heather for being supportive in all my endeavors, making me an overall better person, without you this book wouldn't be possible; to my past and future clients for allowing me to do something I love, because without you this book wouldn't exist. Then, finally, to my parents for showing unconditional love. Thank you for supporting me along the way and for allowing me to chase the things that make me happy.

There are too many more people for me to thank, but I know that everyone who has been a part of my life has helped me get to where I am today, so thank you.

Why This Book Will Change Your Life

Hello, Keegan Brown here. I want to introduce myself and give you an overview of what to expect. Now, most people, when it comes to the word *diet*, they think chicken, rice, and broccoli. Am I right? This book isn't about a diet. It's not going to tell you what to eat, how much, or when. With the concepts in this book, you will have a greater understanding of how to do so. This book is not about a quick, easy solution to your specific goals—muscle mass, strength, or fat loss. However, with what you will learn in this book, you will be able to use these concepts and achieve them.

If you are currently struggling with your diet and it's hard to stick to, you might think it's your fault. Or maybe you're working hard sticking to your diet but aren't seeing the results you want. You're not gaining muscle or losing weight. Maybe you've even stopped progressing, and you don't know why. Or maybe you are a bodybuilder wanting to bring on your best conditioning. This book is about something you can do each and every day. Most books are about losing the most weight as fast as possible. Pick up any book or read any article online, and you will see that most promote easy solutions to much bigger issues. Nutrition is hard. Most diets fail because once they get you to your goal, they don't tell you how you can maintain it or how you can make adjustments. A diet has to go beyond a twenty-one-day fix or an eight-week nutrition program.

In my experience working with a few people, there is good news and bad news. Some of you might read this and never implement anything that's in here. Maybe you've tried dieting multiple times, and you always end up back were you were. Or, if you are a competitor, you may have a postshow rebound and gain back a lot of unwanted body fat.

In order for you to get the most benefit out of this book, you have to have an open mind and forget what you know about dieting. You've been taught over and over again by articles on the Internet, by the media, and maybe even by your family that there are diet foods, and then there are fattening foods. You might be told that you are only allowed to eat clean, healthy foods to reach your goal. I promise that is not something that is sustainable for you to do every day. That can cause cravings and binges that ultimately lead to gaining most of the weight back. In order for you to get the most benefit from this book, you have to be willing to learn and have an open mind, and together we can help fix these problems.

Once you know some of the foundational concepts, we will dive into more complex topics, such as adaptations to dieting, cheat meals/refeed days, gaining insight to the pros and cons of both, and learning how to set them up and how to logically implement them in your diet.

You will learn why you don't have to cut out certain foods from your diet, such as bread, milk, ice cream, or anything else you might enjoy eating, while still getting results you want. You will also learn about metabolic adaptation, the reason why dieting gets harder, and all the implications of it; how to figure out your initial diet; how to maintain all your hard work through reverse dieting; and, ultimately, how this is the only sustainable way to diet, not just for eight weeks, but for LIFE! When you implement all the concepts in this book, you will be able to have a healthy relationship with food, transform your body, and, most importantly, just be happy with yourself.

That is what this book is about.

Introduction

I wanted to write this book not because I'm smarter or better, but mostly because I was once like some of you. Now I'm not saying you are going to compete, but there are a lot of people who have a hard time losing weight or who actually don't know what to do after the diet is over. There are people who would get on a diet and not see results they wanted. Maybe they would lose a little, and then get stressed, binge, and put the weight right back on. Most books or coaches might hand you a diet and tell you to tough it out and trust the process. We all know that you can't stay on low calories forever and eat food you may not necessary like. Personally, after one of my first bodybuilding shows, the show was over, and I was thinking, "What now?"

This book is an accumulation of what I have learned over the years. I have dieted down many times using the same techniques in this book and have had many success stories with clients of mine, online and in person. I don't want you to only view it as a diet book. If you knew you could get in the best shape of your life, what would that do for you?

I hope after reading this book, you will realize that whatever your fitness goal is, whether just to lose a few pounds or to bring your best conditioning to competing, you can achieve it and not have to give up anything you like. It's not going to be a twenty-one-day fix or an eight-week diet. I'm also not going to be the new fitness Instagram model, promoting a new skinny detox drink. Those methods make it seem like fitness is simple, and they *do not* work. You will soon see that this book will provide a ton of value and that reaching your goal is closer than you think.

Different Than Your Typical Diet

When I think of the word *diet*, I think of something not fun and often bland, and I have to eat the same thing every day to get the results I want. In purchasing this book, you have entrusted me with being your coach and helping you. I get that life happens and you sometimes fall off your diet. That's okay because we are all human, and I'm not expecting you to be perfect. Sometimes I fall off my diet, too. I truly appreciate that you are taking the time and reading this book and letting me be a part of your own journey. So how is this book different than a diet?

1. **You will be able to use this plan forever!**
   Science changes all the time, and we are making leaps and bounds when it comes to learning about nutrition. You have probably worked with a coach or nutritionist, or have tried losing weight on your own and failed. That's okay. The concepts I'm going to teach you in this book will never change. They will still apply twenty years from now, even when new studies come out.

2. **I use the same concepts in this book for myself and my clients!**

    There are tons of people teaching the cool new nutrition concepts online and claiming their way of dieting is best. Sometimes you see the new Instagram fitness models promoting a diet or supplement online when they don't use it themselves. Most really don't understand the supplements they are taking in the first place. The thing is, the information in this book really isn't set in stone. You can use this information for gaining muscle, losing fat, or improving sports performance—you name it. These concepts will work. I use them myself and for all my clients (even for contest prep bodybuilding!) Pretty neat, right? I work closely with people online and in person to make them stay on track with nutrition and motivation and to get them in the best shape of their lives. All while eating things they enjoy! Isn't that cool?

3. **Images/Samples**

    I am a visual learner. Throughout this book, you will see images that will make understanding topics a lot easier as we dig deeper into the subject. I'd suggest you read the book from beginning to end and then go back if you get stuck on something. I can't teach you calculus if you skip over learning 2+2. Each topic will build upon the previous topic. If you forget something, you can scroll through the book and look for an image that might help you remember. I'm definitely excited for you to learn and be able to use the concepts in this book. I appreciate your letting me be your coach and a part of your fitness journey!

To Clean or Not to Clean?

The Clean Eating Myth

If you have tried to diet before, you probably know it is hard. You may have snacked on things you were not supposed to, knowing they were bad for you. I know I have done that, even though I knew I was not sticking to a "clean, healthy diet." Those are the terms used to describe a diet, *clean* and *healthy*. Honestly, I'm not even sure what clean means in relation to a diet. I just imagine bodybuilders eating chicken with no seasoning and broccoli from a bowl of Tupperware, trying to hold back the tears as they get a whiff of cheesecake. So what is clean eating? Did you wash your food? Scrub it? Use soap? When you hear the words *healthy* or *clean*, you most certainly think of chicken, rice, vegetables, fruit. You may also think it means getting rid of your sauces, sweets, and even sugar. All the fun stuff, right? For whatever reason, the word *clean* still gets used without a clear meaning.

There are many reasons why I don't like this way of dieting. The first time I remember having some problems with this style of dieting, it was simply life getting in the way. It was about noon, and I was getting ready for one of our family get-togethers. My grandma always makes a couple of special dishes, including pork and beans and our secret family chocolate pie recipe (I won't reveal that in this book, ha-ha!). I don't know how most families are, but the members of my family are very close to one another—everyone from first to third and maybe even fourth cousins. More or less, I have a hard time keeping track of everyone. That day, I was in the middle of preparing for one of my bodybuilding shows, and all I knew was that I couldn't have anything to eat. I spent our entire family outing just imagining what the pie tasted like and trying to decide if having any would be detrimental to my fat loss.

Like most, I know life happens. I like to go out with friends, go to dinner, or just indulge in something delicious, such as ice cream. Maybe you want to take your significant other out on a date, and you just happen to be on this diet. What do you do? I highly doubt you will bring your Tupperware to be filled with tears while you eat your boring meal and smell what's on your date's plate. I have heard some weird stories, such as some people going to the extremes of bringing a food scale to a restaurant. If that's not a way to ruin a date, I don't know what is.

Now, if you are like me, you're not going to bring Tupperware. The truth is, I'm going to go out and enjoy my dinner. The difference between it being okay to enjoy a meal and having it ruin your diet is simple science. Now, if you are a bodybuilder following a more strenuous type of diet to prepare for a show, you might refrain from going out to eat because you have less control over what is served. The biggest issue I normally see with clean eating is having to refrain from eating foods that you enjoy. When I was at our family outing, I really wanted to eat some pie! Now, most people end up starving themselves because they eliminate "bad and unhealthy foods" from their diet, thinking those foods will make them fat and lead to health problems. So how can eating clean or healthy make you fat? Two words—binge eating.

For example, let's say that you are doing well and have eliminated every "bad" food on the planet. The weekend comes around, and you get invited to dinner and there are tons of food options. You find yourself in front of cheeseburgers, fries, sauces, and maybe some brownies. Then what happens? One won't hurt you, right? Only you don't just eat one. You end up eating four or five brownies, a couple of cheeseburgers, and a plate full of fries. In the bodybuilding world, this is known as a cheat day. I know because I have been there.

Most bro diets start by dropping food intake to extremely low levels right off the bat. For some reason, this usually ends up around 1,200 calories per day for women and 1,800 calories per day for the guys. I'm not sure what the logic is behind those numbers. It just seems that's where every clean-diet coach starts, like those numbers have magical fat-loss powers or something. So, what's the biggest problem with doing this? When I think of the word *metabolism,* I find it easiest to define it as reactions in the body. A high metabolism means more reactions in the body, and a low metabolism means fewer reactions in the body.

So, you've been good and have eaten clean and healthy all week. You notice that you initially lost some body fat and feel better about yourself. What happens next? You begin to splurge because you have refrained from eating certain foods. Thus, your metabolism, which is now slow from being in a state of caloric restriction, can't handle the huge amount of food you just ate. This is not a result from the bad food, although this is where most people think the problem lies. The real problem is the result of eating a massive caloric surplus (lots of food) in a short amount of time, when your metabolism is low (few reactions going on). This can be bad for your fat loss diet because you now have just increased your caloric intake way above what you have been used to eating. Guess what happens? All those calories that you just ate will most certainly be stored as body fat if you have not controlled the amount of that intake. People do this for months on end and can't figure out where they messed up. It's not because they ate bad foods; it's because they didn't have guidelines to follow.

Flexible Dieting

As I said previously, you have to have an open mind from here on out before we go any further or this book will be of no value.

So what is flexible dieting? When I think of the word *flexible,* I typically think of something that can bend and twist. Flexible dieting isn't a new concept. You might have heard of it called IIFYM or If It Fits Your Macros, but I don't like those words. I do like the word *flexible*. The biggest misconception is that flexible dieting is all about eating pizza, ice cream, or brownies. Basically, it includes anything you can think of as nondiet foods, right? Well, flexible dieting isn't that. What the name implies is being flexible with your diet. Flexible dieting is mixing and matching foods to hit your overall caloric intake (macronutrients), while still eating enough vitamins, minerals (micronutrients), and daily fiber intake. Your body doesn't know what a clean or healthy food is, but it does know how to metabolize and use it. By hitting your required micronutrients (vitamins and minerals) and fiber (0.2 grams per pound of bodyweight), you can still go eat your pizza, your ice cream, and your favorite kinds of foods while hitting your targeted goal for fitness and health. Then again, flexible dieting isn't a diet. It's also the choice to eat chicken, broccoli, and healthy foods or to eat more filling foods when dieting gets harder.

For example, let's say you are a 150-pound

male or female, and your maintenance calories are roughly around 2,400. Therefore, the recommendation for fiber is around 30 grams (0.2 per pound of bodyweight). With the rest of your calories for the day, you can have some wiggle room. Eat a variety of foods to hit your micronutrient goal first, and then have some of those fun foods you normally wouldn't eat to fill in the macronutrients. Then again, if you are eating around 1,200 calories, there will not be a lot of wiggle room, so then you might choose to eat more filling foods such as rice or broccoli, but you never have to cut out certain foods from your diet.

However, some people will still claim that you need to cut out dairy, gluten, sugar, and processed foods, which is completely false. Unless you have celiac disease, are lactose intolerant, or have some other food allergy, there is no reason to ever eliminate a food from your diet. If you eliminate certain foods and are eating the same thing every day while following a clean eating meal plan, you are more likely to have a deficiency in micronutrients, which will be harmful to your health. You may also be more likely to not follow the diet at all. The only time things can be harmful is like anything else; it's the dosage that will cause negative health effects, not the name of "individual ingredient" because it sounds scary. Think about it in terms of medicine, for example. Read any medication facts label, and it will say to take one or two or no more than a certain amount per day. It will give you a certain dose and also tell you an amount to not go over. For the medication to work, you have to have a minimal effective dose, but there is a dosage at which it can become harmful. So when it comes to food, you never have to eliminate a food item because, it's the dose that becomes harmful. Your body doesn't know a health food from a junk food. What it does know is how to metabolize it and use it.

Why is this great?

This allows you to

1. stick to your daily intake of calories;
2. be flexible and enjoy life;
3. not have a hate relationship with food; and
4. be healthy or improve health. (Yes, you can improve health by eating more delicious things. Bummer, I know.)

REVIEW

You can lose weight eating clean, although it's not practical for long-term success. If you enjoy eating chicken, rice, and broccoli all day, then that is totally okay! That's the joy of flexible dieting—it's your choice! But if you are like most people, clean eating can lead to binge eating. It can make it harder to lose weight from dropping calories to quickly and ultimately set you up for a rebound in weight gain. Life happens, and like me, you probably want to go out with friends, enjoy life, and not have a love/hate relationship with food. That's why flexible dieting is great and is the only sustainable way to diet.

Breaking Down the Science

To really understand the concept of flexible dieting, you have to understand the basics first. You might not fully understand some of the concepts or terminology at first, but that's okay. You will be able to read through this, have an idea of what macro- and micronutrients are, and then be able to use this section to help build your own initial diet. When it comes to dieting, calories are king. There are three macronutrients that make up calories. The big three are protein, carbohydrates, and fats. As we dig deeper into each macronutrient, it's best to learn some of their basic functions. This will help you understand some of the bigger topics later on in this section.

Protein

As soon as you hear the word *protein,* you probably instantly imagine every bodybuilder's favorite macronutrient. It typically is the favorite for a reason. When it comes to any diet, the main focus should be on protein. Protein is what makes up muscle tissue, which is essential for muscle growth. To build muscle, you have to be taking in adequate protein, which will help with muscle protein synthesis (building muscle tissue). It aids in muscle repair, growth, and recovery and can assist in fat loss! Protein can also be a critical fuel source when needed, as your body can break it down to amino acids for energy, although it is very difficult to break down. Out of the three macronutrients, the body has to work the hardest to use protein as energy or to convert it over to fat.

The body can break down proteins into amino acids. After they are broken down, proteins can be absorbed, enter the blood stream, and eventually make their way to muscles and other cells. These amino acids are reassembled to form new muscle tissue. This is how you can get more muscle and become stronger and leaner without sacrificing muscle.

When I first began, I really didn't know where to begin with protein. All I knew was that protein meant muscle and that I had to eat a lot of it. I really didn't understand how much I needed. So, before I knew how much or what actually drove muscle to grow, I was at a sticking point in my diet. I would just eat whatever had protein in it, drinking mass gainer shakes, eating fast food hamburgers, and snacking on anything I thought would help me add size to my 133-pound body frame.

So, you are not alone. Protein is important, but there are also other factors that can help you maintain muscle while on a fat los diet. So, now you know that protein is important because it forms muscle tissue and can aid in fat loss. But how much should you be taking in?

RDA

The current recommendation for the recommended daily allowance (RDA) of protein is 0.8

grams per kilogram of body weight, or basically nothing. The RDA provides these numbers as the recommended minimum amount of protein needed for an individual. This is okay if you wanted to stay inside and watch Netflix all day and never leave the couch. The RDA is for individuals who are not active. The RDA dose is the minimal dose needed to keep a positive nitrogen balance, which is basically the minimum amount of protein needed to maintain muscle tissue if you never left the couch. Since everyone reading this doesn't fit the Netflix scenario and is most likely looking to lose weight, build muscle, or become an athlete, the next section is most likely for you!

The Gold Standard

Now I'm probably going to guess that everyone who has tried to diet, been to a gym, or done a quick Google search has heard of the 1 gram of protein per pound of body weight formula at least one time in their fitness journey. There is a good reason this is the general guideline. It has been shown quite often in research that this will promote muscle growth and aid in fat loss. However, there are also studies that support a lower protein dose of around 0.7–0.8 grams of protein to build and maintain muscle. So where does the 1 gram per pound of bodyweight come from? I believe that people don't like decimal points or math, so rounding to 1 was a good starting point. The question is, can you overdo it?

All the Protein

So, you know that protein is important, and it forms muscle tissue. But do you know how much you should be taking in? Now there have been studies that have shown that you should consume anywhere from 0.7 to 1.5 grams of protein per pound of body weight. In one particular study, the research supported a high protein diet, recommending around 1.5 grams per pound of body weight. Now that is a lot of protein! In that study, participants were given either 1 gram (the gold standard) or 1.5 grams of protein per pound of bodyweight during an eight-week program. Throughout the study, the 1.5 gram per pound of body weight group also consumed about 500 calories per day more than the 1 gram per pound of body weight group. What this study showed was that even though the 1.5 per pound of body weight group had consumed more protein and more calories, both groups had similar muscle gain, but the 1.5 gram per pound group lost more body fat! Now I'm not saying, "Yea! Eat all the protein!" I will teach you how to utilize this information later on. However, another thing people miss is how to maximize this intake through muscle protein synthesis.

Muscle Protein Synthesis

Besides understanding the right amount of protein you should consume, I believe understanding muscle protein synthesis (MPS) is just as important. Not all the protein you eat becomes muscle tissue. Muscle protein synthesis is the signaling of proteins to become muscle tissue. This will play a role in keeping muscle while on a fat loss diet or will even help build muscle tissue more optimally.

Now if you are like most people, including me, you probably read every single label and add up every little bit of protein, from the 25 grams you got from chicken to the less than 1 gram you got from some drink. I used to get home, start cooking food, open the fridge, and read labels. By the time I added everything up, I would have three to four different sources of protein to make up something around 25–30 grams. The problem with this was that none of those separate protein sources was causing a great enough anabolic response (the signal to build muscle). So how do you go about signaling muscle protein synthesis?

There is no definitive answer as to the maximum amount of protein that is really beneficial at a meal, although there is some research that has been shown to be helpful. That research deals with the amino acid leucine, which is one of the biggest drivers of MPS. Leucine is an amino acid responsible for triggering an anabolic response, and different protein sources have been shown to elicit anabolic responses in proportion to the amount of leucine they contain. So the more leucine you consume, the stronger the signal for muscle to grow. Now here is the bigger question—how much leucine do you need?

Although there has been research done, it appears that consuming approximately 0.02 grams of leucine per pound of bodyweight at a meal will maximize your anabolic response to that protein source. This would be about 3–4 grams of leucine for the average person.

For example, if you were a two-hundred-pound person, you would be aiming for around 3–4 grams of leucine per meal. So, for a high-leucine protein source like whey, which contains roughly 12 percent leucine, you would require about 30–35 grams of protein from whey to max out anabolism and cause the greatest amount of muscle protein synthesis to occur. From something like casein, which is slow to digest and has lower amounts of leucine of around 8 percent, you would need to eat around 50 grams of protein to have the same MPS benefit.

Review

Out of the three macronutrients, I consider protein the most important. That does not mean you should neglect the other two. I was actually under eating on some days going into my competition, and I actually lost a lot of muscle tissue preparing for my competition. The biggest reason for this was that I wasn't as consistent with eating the same amounts of protein each day, and I also neglected the MPS response from eating smaller meals. While eating my clean diet, I ate about four meals a day, while trying to get leaner and work around my school schedule. I lost fat but also lost muscle in the process. Being consistent and eating the right amount of protein each day will help you keep hard earned muscle and aid in fat loss.

Fats

I remember watching an episode of *Seinfeld*, about the time back in the 1980s when a lot of people thought fat was bad and eating it would make you fat. The characters would sit around this ice cream parlor and just eat everything that contained zero fat. They would buy fat free ice cream and fat free yogurts, but they actually ended up gaining weight because of it. So what gives?

When it comes to fat, fats are not the enemy. Fats won't make you fat unless you overconsume them, putting you in a caloric surplus (eating more than what your body is using for fuel). You can also have too little fat and end up with aching joints, decreased testosterone and decreased performance. However, if you overconsume fat, it can easily be stored as body fat.

There are different kinds of fats that have different benefits. So, before we can best utilize them, we have to understand how they are used. I'm not going to talk about every single one, but the most common fats that I get asked about are polyunsaturated fats (specifically omega-3s), saturated fats, and trans fats.

Omega-3s

Omega-3 fats usually do get associated with the healthy fats. These have been shown to help aching joints, aide in recovery, and increase fat loss by turning on certain genes. These can be found in things such as tuna, salmon, and fish oils (so, mostly fish).

Saturated Fats

Now these usually get a bad report mostly because people associate them with coronary heart disease, cardiovascular disease, and cholesterol. Saturated fats are generally looked at by most people as bad. When it comes to High Density Lipoproteins (HDL cholesterol) and Low Density Lipoproteins (LDL cholesterol), HDL is considered to be good, while LDL is considered to be bad. HDL is shown to be a transporter of LDL from the blood stream back to the liver, while LDL is usually associated with plaque buildup in the arteries.

Trans-fats

When it comes to all the fats, these are the only ones that don't really provide any benefit besides being an energy source. Trans fats are usually associated with cholesterol (LDL), coronary heart disease, and cardiovascular disease.

So keep omega-3 fats, avoid saturated fats, and don't even look at trans fats then. Got it? Well, no...

Like most of you, when I was first learning about science, I learned about the scientific method. Basically, to conduct an experiment, you have to have a control group, independent variable (something that doesn't change), and a dependent variable (something you change). Maybe you recall that or you don't, but this is where a lot of studies possibly mess up early on. In order to compare fats to one another, you can't have changes in other macronutrients (proteins and carbohydrates), and you also have to match equal fat intake.

For example, if you were eating 150 grams of protein, 80 grams of fat, and 100 grams of carbohydrate, you have to keep the protein, carbohydrate, and fat calorie content equal. The only thing you change is the source, going from a saturated to polyunsaturated fat and keeping them at 80 grams of fat.

So what really happens when you do control the amount of fat calories and then compare them? When comparing saturated fats to unsaturated fats (polyunsaturated or monounsaturated), the saturated fat didn't negatively affect heart health. But when people did consume a poly or monounsaturated fat, it did tend to improve heart health. Now you're probably wondering what that really means. That means that, when controlled, there tends to be a weak correlation between dietary saturated fats and cardiovascular disease or coronary heart disease. Cool, right?

Cholesterol

You might have head of things like eggs, being high in saturated fats, are bad for you because they affect LDL cholesterol levels. However, when they looked at dietary cholesterol, dietary cholesterol from saturated fats had a weak correlation between dietary and blood cholesterol. Correlation doesn't mean causation. Dietary cholesterol is not responsible for blood cholesterol.

In other words, consuming saturated fats compared to consuming unsaturated fats (when controlled) didn't affect health negatively, and dietary cholesterol from saturated fats had a weak correlation between dietary and blood cholesterol. When they compared both equally and substituted a saturated for an unsaturated, health improved. That means you don't have to get rid of any type of fat. When controlled, they won't affect you negatively. Negative health risks don't arise because of the type of fat. What you should look at is how much you are eating. So what about trans fats? As you read earlier, it's pretty much only good for energy or fat storage. When we compare fats equally, trans fats won't cause negative health risks if controlled, but they can't offer any benefit besides energy. I would limit trans fats, but you don't have to eliminate them from your diet.

Testosterone

Most people associate the word *testosterone* with muscle! This is with good reason, as it can aid in muscle repair and promote fat loss. When thinking in terms of fats, research has shown that an increase in saturated fats actually increases testosterone levels. Now this doesn't mean you can go all crazy. The proportion of testosterone for muscle isn't linear. So having more testosterone doesn't mean you will pack on more muscle, even though I wish it did. If you are dieting, you might consider taking in some forms of saturated fats because when you diet, hormone levels tend to decrease.

Review

Fats won't make you fat like they thought in the episode of *Seinfeld*. They can help with a lot of things from joints, testosterone, and cholesterol. I don't want you to see saturated fats as bad and omega-3 fats as good. I will say to limit trans-fats, but there is no need to get rid of any of them. Yes, even trans fats! When comparing saturated to unsaturated fat, neither posed any health risks. This also goes for cholesterol and heart health. When looking at fats, don't see them just as good and bad. Look at fats and ask what benefits they have. And, remember that a specific type of fat won't make you fat, but overconsumption will.

Carbohydrates

Carbohydrates are probably the most underrated macronutrient. Practically everyone thinks you can just look at carbohydrates and—poof—you gain body fat! But, carbohydrates actually can be protein sparing, meaning they can help preserve muscle, aid in energy, and reduce the amount of protein you need to eat.

Therefore, carbohydrates are critical to include in your diet.

For instance, if you are in a caloric deficit (expending more energy than you are consuming), your body might try to turn those amino acids into glucose, which is another reason to have enough protein in your diet, especially while focusing on fat loss. Your body can produce enough carbohydrates (glucose), mainly in your liver, from the protein and fat you consume. This does *not* mean to get rid of carbohydrates or to eat extremely low amounts of them.

Carbohydrates can help prevent breakdown of proteins and fats because they can be easily broken down and used as glucose, thereby sparing protein and amino acids from oxidation (burning/being used for fuel). During exercise, they can be muscle sparing as well, especially during heavy compound exercises.

Glycemic Index

You probably have heard some person tell you that, when dieting, you can't have donuts, candy, fruit, or anything really sugary. I have been told that, and I still hear it a lot whether reading an article online or talking to a bodybuilder walking around the gym only eating chicken, rice, and sweet potatoes for every meal of the day. So how does this play into the glycemic Index?

The glycemic index is more or less just a number associated with a type of carbohydrate and related to how it impacts blood glucose (sugar) levels. So you can have a food on the low end of the scale such as rice (low glycemic) or something high on the scale such as Kool-Aid (high glycemic).

One day, I overheard someone say that you can't have sugar in your diet because it can make you fat. The reason he gave was that insulin is the fat storage hormone. Yes, that might be the definition you will read in a book. However, there was a study done that compared high-glycemic to low-glycemic diets in obese men and women. They had three different groups (a high-glycemic-index group, a low-glycemic-index group, and a low-fat-diet group). The diets consisted of 3,138 kilojoules less than estimated energy needs (being in a slight caloric deficit). When comparing the groups together in a controlled caloric intake, what they found was that the groups had shown no differences. I thought that was awesome, but what does that actually tell us?

The study indicates that if you were eating 200 grams of carbohydrates, and most of those came from something like rice (low glycemic), you could substitute something like gummy bears (high glycemic), if you control the number of calories consumed.

Insulin and Fat Loss

Now, you're probably thinking a little since I just told you that you can have sugar on a fat loss diet. One of the things probably rambling through your mind is insulin since I just told you about glycemic index. As you know, you typically think of insulin as the almighty fat storage hormone because it takes glucose (sugar) from your bloodstream and stores it. I believe, when thinking in terms of fat loss, this is one of the most misunderstood concepts. People usually end up eating some low carb diet or low-glycemic foods such as rice because they think any insulin is bad for fat loss.

For fat loss to occur, you have to release fatty acids into the bloodstream (lipolysis). However, if you don't use it, it can also go back into storage (lipogenesis). Fat burning is blunted by insulin, but it's not shut down. Fat burning (oxidation) is a twenty-four-hour process. All these processes are all going on at once, so if you are in a calorie surplus, the rate at which it's being stored is faster than the rate at which it's being released or burned. If you are in a deficit, the rate at which it's being released and burned is greater than the rate at which it is being stored. Just like anything else, it depends on the concentration. Assuming calories are equal, if you have high amounts of insulin in one meal by eating something sugary, you will make up for it by having lower insulin responses the rest of the day, because it's a twenty-four-hour process. Now, as mentioned earlier when referring back to the glycemic index, when comparing a low-glycemic to a high-glycemic diet, studies found no differences with improved insulin sensitivity! Well, you might ask, what does that actually mean?

I like to think of insulin as a string. (Go get a string if you have one.) The middle of the string represents the degree of an insulin response. The ends of the string represent how long it takes for insulin to come back down.

Let's say you have a three-foot-long string, and you hold it end to end. If controlled, that string will always be three feet in length. While the length will always be the same, the distance of the ends might be closer or farther apart depending on how much you pull on the middle of it.

Now grab the middle of the string. If you were to eat something like rice (low glycemic), you might have a low insulin response. Now pick up the middle of the string slightly. The string is still three feet long, but the ends of the string move a little closer together. Now, let's say you end up eating something like a candy bar (high glycemic). Pick up the middle of the string and pull it really high. What you notice is that the string is still three feet long, but the ends of the string come a lot closer together.

So, in the first scenario, you barely picked up the middle of the string. This indicates a very small increase in insulin and that it also takes a lot longer for insulin to come back down. In the second scenario, you picked up the middle of the string again but pulled on it a lot more. In this case, the insulin comes crashing back down a lot faster. Therefore, if controlled, the amount of insulin will be the same, but how long it takes for insulin to come back down might be different. However, the string will be the same length, no matter how much of an insulin response you have.

Another comparison that I like is mail delivery. Imagine taking mail (food) to the mailbox. The mailman comes by and picks it up (insulin) and takes it away to the post office (storage). Now imagine you have no mail to put in the mailbox. When the mailman comes by, he won't be able to deliver anything to the post office. That means if you are in a calorie deficit, insulin won't have an impact on your fat loss.

Review

Carbohydrates are probably the most underrated of the three macronutrients. The key thing I want you to take away from this is that carbohydrates are not the enemy. They can aid in keeping muscle while you are on a fat loss diet, and carbohydrates alone are not going to pack on the pounds. As you now know, you can eat whatever type of carbohydrates you like because the glycemic index doesn't matter. There may be more optimal times to enjoy treats, such as candy bars or your favorite dessert, but those things won't make you fat so you never have to cut them out completely from your diet!

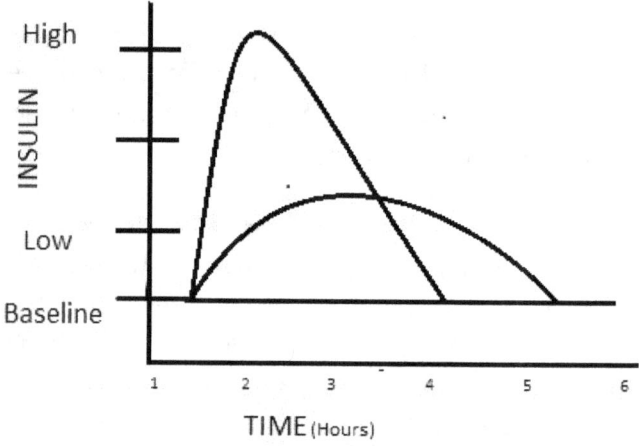

Micronutrients

If I say the word *micronutrients*, you probably think of vitamins and minerals, alongside fruits and vegetables. People who don't understand flexible dieting usually don't understand the basics of eating a variety of foods. Is it logical to think you will get all your vitamins and minerals by eating the same foods every day? Now, I'm not saying my entire diet consists of hamburgers. Yes, you do have to eat some fruits and vegetables, but if you go into your fridge right now and pick up a box of cereal, I guarantee they have vitamins and minerals in them. Instead of just thinking fruits and vegetables all day, learn to read a label, and you might be surprised about how many micronutrients are in foods you consider to be bad.

Review

Whether or not you really understood everything I just said, that's okay. The whole point of this section was to show what the macronutrients are, to discuss their additional benefits (besides being fuel for your body), and to tell you that you can have things that are considered bad for you. Remember the study that compared saturated fats to unsaturated fats and found no negative effect on health. If you take one thing away from this section, I want you to realize that nutrition isn't and shouldn't be a one-size-fits-all thing. You don't have to eat chicken, broccoli, and rice all day. It's 100 percent okay to eat things you enjoy! The beautiful thing called science says so. I know you will go out and enjoy yourself at restaurants, go to dinners and movies, or even eat things like chocolate pies. That's just life. I want you to know that one thing isn't going to be the reason why you can't lose weight. When controlled and when everything else is matched calorie for calorie, you can have anything and not have to worry about it making you fat.

Building Your Initial Diet

At the very beginning of this book, I said that this will be different than your typical diet because this is not a diet. This book won't tell you what to eat. In order to be sustainable, your diet should be composed of foods you actually enjoy eating, right? It's not going to be bland chicken, broccoli, and rice eaten from Tupperware unless that's stuff you really like.

The truth is you don't have to eat the same thing every day. If you made it this far and I didn't bore you, that's great! The rest of this section is about building something you can use. Whether you are a stay-at-home parent, someone with a busy work schedule and you have to eat out more often then you should, or a competitive bodybuilding athlete, this section is for you. This is where I start with my clients and with myself. The cool thing is that you will be building your own diet. I'll show you how to set up a personalized plan for yourself.

If you've been on a diet before, it was probably something like the following:

MEAL 1:   ¼ oatmeal , 4 egg whites, 1 yolk

MEAL 2:   4 ounces chicken, 1 cup veggies

Meal 3:   3 egg whites, 1 tbs almond butter

I've worked with people who have come to me with a diet similar to the one above. This is actually a former diet of one of my clients from a previous coach. What's the problem with this?

If you have had something similar to the diet above, you will have no idea if you will be gaining weight, losing weight, or staying the same. Granted this is a very small amount of food to begin with, you will learn later why this is bad to start with later on in the book, but how do you go about making adjustments to this plan? All your body knows is how to metabolize. Food is fuel.

The most important part of dieting isn't the quality of food—it's the quantity. Whether you end up eating 1 cup of brown rice or choosing some other carbohydrate source such as cereal, all your body knows to do is how to use it. It will break those carbohydrates down to sugar to be used as fuel or to be stored as body fat. Your body doesn't know what a 100 percent free-range, organic hamburger is. Once you start seeing food as a fuel source, dieting gets a little easier.

Starting Calories

If you've been online and looked at calorie counters, there are a ton of them to choose from, but none are going to be accurate. They might be a ballpark estimate, but none really tell you what your current maintenance calories are. The only way to truly figure out what your maintenance calories needs are and your current metabolic rate is, is to track your calories for a period of five to seven days and get an average. If you are not gaining or losing weight, this will be the number of calories to which your metabolism has adjusted. For instance, let's say you found you were consuming an average of around 1,500 calories a day, but the calculator you found online says you could consume around 1,900 calories per day and lose weight. That would be around 400 calories more per day than you have been consuming on average. In reality, you might put body fat back on if you followed what the calculator indicated. If you don't want to track right off the bat, you can use the calculator to get close. From there you can make adjustments.

There are many online sources where you can log what you eat for the next five to seven days, such as myfitnesspal.com. This site provides one of the closest estimates available for accurate calorie intake, and it is what I usually use with my own clients. For myself, I like to use pen and paper and just write everything down.

Starting Macronutrients

Once you figure out starting calories, you can figure out your starting macronutrient needs (protein, carbohydrate, and fat). Earlier, I discussed their importance and how they make up total calories. If you have already been doing this that great! You just have a head start.

1 gram of protein has 4 calories

1 gram of fat has 9 calories

1 gram of carbohydrate has 4 calories

For example, if you eat thirty grams of protein,

ten grams of fat, and twenty grams of carbohydrate, that would equal 290 calories.

4 calories from proteins x 30 g = 120 calories

9 calories from fats x 10 g = 90 calories

4 calories from carbohydrates x 20 g = 80 calories

Total for this meal would be 290 calories.

Each meal that you have eaten throughout the day adds up to your total daily calorie intake. Although it is important to eat all the calories for the day, it's also important to balance out each meal to support energy throughout the day. For the sake of building a sample diet, I'm going to use a 150-pound person as an example and going to assume he has figured his maintenance calorie needs to be 2,300. Recall that protein is what drives muscle growth, aids in fat loss, and is used as energy as needed. When initially figuring out protein amounts, I start with 1 gram per pound of body weight. 1 gram per pound of body weight is enough to promote a positive nitrogen balance, support muscle protein synthesis, and aid in fat loss. However, if you are someone who has more body fat to lose, you might start with 0.7 grams of protein per pound of body weight.

For example, if you are a person who weighs 280 pounds and has more than 30 percent of body fat to lose, you would calculate your protein needs as follows:

0.7 x 280 = 196 g of protein

For most people, the cheapest and easiest way to determine body fat percentage is by going to your local gym and getting a caliper test or doing a handheld electrical impedance test. Are they 100 percent accurate? No, but either of these tests will give you a really good estimate and will be a great starting point.

When it comes to nutrition and fat loss, fat intake is one of the bigger hormonal regulators in the body. If you eat too little fat, you get decreased testosterone, aching joints and decreased performance. Too much dietary fat can easily be stored as body fat. Research has shown that going below 15 percent of total calories dedicated to fat decreased test levels. While I am not saying go all out and eat all the fat as it can easily be stored as body fat, I usually start between 0.3–0.5 grams of fat per pound of body weight.

So if you are a 150-pound person, your protein intake would be around 150 grams, while your fat intake will be between 45–75 grams. I usually go on the lower side of fat intake as I like my carbohydrates, but if I start to get aching joints, I might increase it using the 0.5 per pound marker. Then, the rest of the calories will come from carbohydrates.

So, if you are a 150-pound person, your total

will be around 150 grams of protein, 45 grams of fat, and then you can figure out carbohydrates using simple subtraction to figure out what calories are left over. This leaves us with the following calculation:

Protein 150 g x 4 calories = 600

Fats 45 g x 9 calories = 405

Carbohydrates 324 g x 4 calories = 1,295 (rounded from 323.75 carbohydrates)

Now that you have figured out what your initial calories are and what your initial macronutrients are, its best to spread these out to support energy. For example, if you typically have five meals per day, each meal might include 30 grams protein, 9 grams fat, and 65 grams carbohydrate. Remember, this is just an example.

I like to eat four to five meals per day. If you recall from the protein section and the discussion of muscle protein synthesis, this will help with muscle growth. It's best to make these meals and days consistent. If you miss one meal and then snack, it might be hard to make up macronutrients or calories later in the day. Also, these should come from foods you actually enjoy. So, if you want to eat egg whites, ham, toast, honey, and orange juice for meal one and then eat chicken and rice for meal two, that is totally fine. For meal three, you might try to add in some ice cream or whatever suits your taste buds and allows you to stick to something long term.

Overall, you should take five to seven days and figure out how many calories you have been eating on average. You can even track macronutrients if you want to during the five to seven days as well. That's what I like to do personally. Once you find an average, you can make the adjustments based on my recommendations as a starting point when making an initial diet from maintenance calories. Once you figure out the macronutrients and overall calories, divide them into four to six meals spread throughout the day, using foods you enjoy. Before we get into how to make changes as you progress, you should know some of the reasoning behind why dieting gets hard and learn about some of the adaptations that occur through dieting so you have an understanding what's going on.

Metabolic Adaptation

When flexible dieting first came around, there were a lot of things for which we actually didn't have a name for. Before the term metabolic adaptation, initially it was called *metabolic damage*. When that term spread, a lot of people got mad at their coaches, trainers, and nutritionists, believing they were damaging their metabolisms. However, you really don't damage a metabolism. What happens is that it changes.

Metabolism can change so much that even if you have body fat to lose, you might have to spend a time eating a surplus of food and building a metabolism just so you can create a deficit for fat loss to occur. This can make fat loss seem nearly impossible because things such as adaptive thermogenesis and hormones that ultimately favor decreased energy expenditure are making you hungrier and decreasing overall satiety.

As phases of a diet progress, this makes fat loss really difficult, despite eating low amounts of food and doing high amounts of exercise. Following calorie restriction and high amounts of exercise, adaptations can results in rapid weight regain after slight calorie increases.

There are some common misconceptions about metabolic adaptation, such as it can make weight loss impossible. Basically, these adaptations are not some magical thing holding you back from losing body fat, but they can make it harder, especially if you are starting with a lot of weight training ,and cardio and are eating like a baby rabbit. It will make it harder to increase energy expenditure or to keep decreasing food. That could pose health risks and is no longer practical. Then again, if you didn't have these kinds of adaptations, weight loss would be super easy and actually make the body more susceptible to starving, still posing a health risk.

For example, if you didn't have these adaptations and your current metabolic rate was around 3,200 calories and you dropped your caloric intake down to 2,600, eventually you would starve yourself off on a 2,600-calorie diet.

Another misconception is that you've followed an improper diet. Like you now know, not one food will make you fat or make it harder to lose weight. It's more about improper dieting rather than the diet itself.

Like I said earlier, your body is more or less just a bunch of ongoing chemical reactions. Recall that a higher metabolism means more reactions in the body and that a low metabolism means fewer reactions. Therefore, if you drop calories too quickly and do excessive amounts of cardio, when your metabolic rate adjusts to your new calories and you still have fat mass to lose, then you have to either keep lowering calories or increasing energy expenditure. Do you see where this can be a problem?

If you start with super low calories, you have to keep dropping calories from 1,200 to lose body fat. Then you are left trying to figure out if you can actually add in any more exercise. If you can make small adjustments over time so you are eating more and doing minimal cardio, you will have a lot more variables available later on when dieting might get harder.

Metabolism

I'm not going to go into super detail about metabolism. If I did that you might just be overwhelmed and put the book down, unless you just love science. My goal is to give you an overview of things you can do with a little understanding as to why you are doing them and not just taking my word for it.

Metabolic Rate

Your metabolic rate is determined by a lot of different factors such as basal metabolic rate (BMR). Remember the Netflix scenario from earlier on in the book? BMR is basically the minimal amount of energy needed to run your bodily systems. You have nonexercise activity thermogenesis (NEAT), which is the fancy way of describing exercise that is not truly exercise, such as walking from your parked car into work. There is also exercise activity thermogenesis

(EAT), such as going to the gym and exercising for an hour.

Then lastly there is the thermic effect of food (TEF), which is basically the amount of energy required to break down food, absorb it, and eventually use it. More or less, when you eat a pizza, your body figures out how much total energy to expend to use that pizza for bodily processes.

All these—BMR, NEAT, EAT, and TEF—make up your total daily energy expenditure (TDEE). Your metabolic rate is forever changing, with a fat loss goal your total daily energy expenditure, TDEE has been shown to consistently decrease over time. This metabolic rate decrease from TDEE is also known as adaptive thermogenesis.

Adaptive Thermogenesis

Remember TDEE includes everything such as BMR, NEAT, EAT, and TEF. All these change, even BMR. Exercise activity thermogenesis decreases as weight decreases. This means that tasks gets easier for your body to do. Maybe you start running when you weigh 200 pounds. You lose some weight and now you weigh 170 pounds. Now, that particular task is easier for you to accomplish. With weight decreases, NEAT energy expenditure goes down. For example, your normal walk into work from the parking lot got easier because you've lost a little bit of body weight. Now, you don't have to expend as much energy to walk. Thermic effect of food changes as well although you won't expend less energy actually digesting, absorbing, or metabolizing. You are expending less total energy digesting, absorbing, and metabolizing indirectly because overall food intake is lowered. You have a total decrease in total calories.

Hormones and Eating Less

There are multiple hormones that regulate body composition and have an effect on metabolic adaptation. I want to highlight a few of them, especially triiodothyronine and thyroxine from the thyroid gland, also known as T3, and T4. In short, if you have higher amounts of circulating T3 and T4, you will have an increased metabolic rate. And if you have low T3 and T4, you will have a lower metabolic rate. The cool thing is that although the thyroid hormones are important, they usually won't be of concern unless you have hypothyroidism, as T3 and T4 are tightly regulated by the thyroid gland. If that is a problem, it will have to be controlled. Otherwise, it will make weight loss harder. Two other hormones that play an important role in metabolism are leptin and ghrelin. Leptin, a hormone found in adipose tissue, can also make fat loss harder. Leptin is an indicator of energy availability. Thus, a higher body fat level means more leptin and is associated with increased energy expenditure and increased satiety (fullness), while lower body fat levels mean lower amounts of leptin. Ghrelin, another hormone, functions to stimulate food intake and ultimately makes you feel hungrier.

There are tons of studies out there that show when you are eating at a calorie deficit, thyroid hormones go down, leptin goes down, and ghrelin goes up. Basically metabolism goes down, leptin is signaling that you don't have energy to use, and ghrelin is telling you to go look in your fridge. These hormones are made to preserve normal body fat levels and will also be elevated throughout a diet while you trying to lose weight. So what can you do about it?

Practical Applications

You now know there are multiple things that affect your metabolic rate. On a fat loss diet, there are multiple changes that occur that are geared to preserve energy and keep body fat. Earlier, I used an example of eating 1,200 calories. In that example, when metabolic rate adjusts to your new calories and you still have fat mass to lose, you have to either keep dropping calories or increase energy expenditure.

Therefore, it is recommended to use the smallest amount of changes to get results. Fat loss and even muscle mass should be seen as a step-by-step process. Fat loss is not a straight line as most of you know. Neither is putting on muscle mass. As you begin a diet, weight loss plateaus will happen. The next logical step would be to change caloric intake or increase energy expenditure to keep creating new deficits as metabolism adjusts.

Refeeding versus Cheat Meals

Nutritionally, there are some things you can do that relate to the hormone leptin. As you now know, leptin is one of primary energy hormones that regulate expenditure. When leptin levels are higher, your body will favor increased energy expenditure and when they are low they will favor a slower metabolism. Leptin levels are highly correlated with the level of carbohydrate intake. If leptin is low, ghrelin will be higher and, as you know, ghrelin will try to make you go back to the fridge to see if you have any snacks—ha ha! Therefore, overeating is beneficial.

There are two ways people usually go about this. I know throughout the bodybuilding world, it has become a norm to hear the term *cheat meal* or my preferred word, *refeed*. Overall, both describe an overeating period that can usually last from one to two days, and that's mostly made up of carbohydrates because higher carbohydrates have been associated with increased leptin levels.

The purpose is to increase circulating levels of leptin and stimulate metabolic rate to increase energy expenditure. As you know, your BMR, NEAT, EAT, TEF, and hormones such as T3, T4, and leptin all begin to slow down the longer you are in a calorie deficit. If your body thinks it's on the brink of starvation, it will do anything to bring fat loss to a halt. Your body does not favor fat loss. So, what you should do is work with its own metabolic adaptations.

You might have heard of a cheat meal if you have ever followed a clean-eating type of diet as you are overeating on purpose to stimulate leptin to increase expenditure. In the clean eating world, this is the norm. You restrict yourself to just eating clean food, and then you get to binge for one day. The problem with this is that if you have been dieting for a period of time, your metabolic rate is slow.

It would be quite easy to overeat on calories and gain more than a little bit of unwanted body fat back. So, I am not an advocate of cheat days whatsoever. But there are some slight benefits of a cheat meal. It does allow you to take a break from tracking if you don't go on a full-out binge and if you are conscious about what you eat. I will personally do this when im trying to put on muscle mass, and weight. I wouldn't do this for a fat loss type diet. If you do end up doing a cheat meal, the last thing I want you to do is feel guilty. This will more likely make you do something bizarre, such as not eat that much the next day or drastically increase cardio to try to compensate. Your bodily system doesn't work like that for fat loss.

Another thing you should do is be consistent. If you have them too close together, it can be easily stored, and you might just be bouncing along through a vicious cycle of losing a small amount of weight followed by gaining it back after each cheat meal.

Now, if you follow some form of flexible dieting or count macronutrients (even if it's a chicken, broccoli, and rice diet), you more information than just a guess on how much you can have. That's why I prefer refeed days. For one, I don't eliminate anything from my diet or any of my clients' diets either. From a logical standpoint, I don't know why you have to eat clean all the time but are allowed to eat bad foods or binge once a week? Like that makes total sense, right?

Refeed days are a more scientific approach to overfeeding. If you do follow flexible dieting or track macronutrients, you know how much you are eating. You have guidelines to follow and are not cheating if you normally eat those foods anyway. Since this is more of a systematic approach, you are less likely to overshoot as compared to a cheat meal or cheat day. Another benefit of a refeed day is to replenish glycogen, the storage form of carbohydrates. The longer you are on a diet, and as you keep making adjustments, you might notice energy plummeting on certain days or overall. An overeating type day will allow you to replenish glycogen so you can keep training harder

A general recommendation to use for a refeed day is to not feel guilty. Just like a cheat day, nothing will make you fall of track more than feeling guilty. This will make you overcompensate somehow through cardio, eat less the next day, or mentally quit all together. This is a more scientific approach to food intake. Therefore, it is wise to stay as close as possible to your amounts of protein, carbohydrates, and fats. As I said earlier, leptin is highly correlated to carbohydrate intake. So, I suggest not changing protein or fat amounts. This will help out with overeating by minimizing potential fat gain and making it easier overall to track for a refeed type day. So how many carbohydrates should your refeed day consist of?

Throughout writing this book, the whole point was to make it evergreen, meaning these concepts will apply to everyone who reads them, whether you're a competitive bodybuilder or someone wanting to lose a few pounds. So, something to consider when figuring out a refeed type day is what are you currently eating now. If you are eating about 300 grams of carbohydrates a day and losing body fat, I'm not going to tell you to go overboard and eat 600 grams or more. You may not need a refeed day at all. It will also depend on how depleted you are and your energy levels.

A general starting point and my recommendation is around 0.5 multiplied by your current carbohydrate intake, or roughly 3 times your body weight. So, if you are dieting off of 300 grams of carbohydrates and a 150 pound person, a refeed day would be about 450 grams. These are not set in stone numbers, but a good starting point. Now, what's your current body fat percentage? If you have a higher body fat percentage of around 30 percent or more, you may not need a refeed day. But if you are someone around 10 percent body fat or trying to get down into the single digits, you can use a refeed day or refeed days. Generally, the leaner you get, the more refeed days you can incorporate into your diet. So, instead of doing the example of 450 grams of carbohydrates for one refeed day, you might do maintenance carbohydrates of 300 grams for two refeed days. Remember, leptin is a hormone found in adipose tissue. Generally, the higher your body fat percentage, the higher the circulating levels of leptin you have. And a lower percentage of body fat indicates lower levels of leptin.

Once you actually start incorporating a refeed day, you can usually adjust it to make it fit your needs. Using 300 grams of carbohydrates as an example again, if you are a male and incorporate a refeed day of 450 grams of carbohydrates and end up losing 5 pounds, this might be too fast and you might try raising your total carbohydrates a little or increasing your refeed days. Then again, if you are not losing fast enough, maybe only half a pound or less, then you might decrease the total carbohydrates or decrease your number of refeed days. When it comes to dieting, rate of loss (ROL) is important. If you diet too fast, you might cause your metabolism to slow. On the other hand, you want to drop it fast enough to actually make progress. A general effective ROL is around one to two pounds a week.

One thing I do notice is some diet coaches recommending six days of super low-calorie intake followed by a super high-calorie cheat day, all with tons of cardio. They just keep that plan in place for twelve weeks. That's what one of my clients went through with someone else. Sometimes maybe not even a cheat day.

While a lot of coaches make it seem to be something magical, the truth is it doesn't increase metabolic rate that much at all, only around 7 percent. You might wind up putting body fat back on because of the untracked cheat meals and by eating lower amounts of carbohydrates throughout the week. Not to mention you might feel awful.

If you are a competitor, this is probably something you don't want to do while trying to reach extremely low percent body fat levels and trying to keep as much muscle mass as possible. If you can keep carbohydrate intake higher throughout the week and incorporate a smaller refeed type day or days, that would be a little better, not just for your metabolism but for your energy as well.

Cardio for Optimal Fat Loss

As I said earlier, you may want to reduce calorie intake or increase energy expenditure to keep creating new deficits as your metabolism adjusts. The next logical step would be to increase energy expenditure through cardio. Before I get into cardio, you should understand that cardio is like the basic screwdriver in your tool box. The main goals of fat loss should be to preserve muscle and lose body fat. Yes, every kind of cardio will work for fat loss, but you should ask yourself which type is optimal, and what is right for you? In this section I break it down if you are looking for general fat loss, or if you are a competitor looking to retain as much muscle mass as possible.

Fat burning is not an immediate process. In order to lose body fat, you have to release it from the cells (lipolysis) and use it as fuel (oxidation), otherwise known as fat burning. Most people think in terms of how much fat they burned during their workouts. What you really should be looking at is how much fat you burned over the course of the day. Now, there are different types of cardio that can be used throughout training. This is not a one size fits all category, but if the goal is fat loss, you want to keep mass while losing body fat. There are different kinds of cardio that use different energy sources as primary fuel during exercise. Two of the most common forms are low intensity steady state (LISS) and high intensity interval training (HIIT).

Walk into any gym around and you will probably see one or more people doing some form of low intensity steady state cardio. This is more or less walking or jogging without changing speed. The primary advantage of doing LISS is that it is safer for the joints and uses fat as its primary fuel source. Now, most of you do cardio before or after you work out with weights. If you do it before your workout, you could impact energy levels. Doing it after your workout, could decrease the muscle protein synthesis response from training.

The other primary cardio you may see, and you may often see it performed wrong, is high intensity interval training. This type of workout is hard. How many people do you see doing full-out sprints as fast as they can go? Or doing battling ropes as hard as they can?

Now I am a big advocate of HIIT for more than one reason for non-contest athletes. One advantage is that it's much shorter in duration. How long can you run at your most optimal speed? If you are lucky, you can full-out sprint for maybe around fifteen seconds, probably less. Generally, HIIT can include anywhere from three to seven sprint intervals. Personally I am dead after about five. So if you ran seven times for fifteen seconds each, then you have 105 seconds of total all-out sprints. If you were doing steady state type cardio, you could be in there for over an hour. Another advantage is that HIIT will signal muscle protein synthesis. It will signal muscle to grow. When compared to low intensity cardio, HIIT keeps your metabolic rate elevated longer postcardio. It also increases mitochondrial and enzyme production. Why is that great? Glad you asked!

As of a result of more mitochondrial and enzyme production, you increase the capacity at which fat can be oxidized (burned). This does not occur in LISS type workouts. This means fat burning will be elevated longer throughout the day after a HIIT workout.

So, great! I will just do HIIT seven days a week, and I will just get super lean! Well, no. The down side of doing HIIT is that it is very taxing to your system. HIIT is basically a continuation of weight training to some degree. Imagine having a training program five days a week and doing HIIT every day? Most likely you will crash and burn halfway through, and that will affect your weight training, which will not be good. So is there a place for doing low intensity steady state cardio?

Although it doesn't provide any metabolic benefit, the main purpose of low intensity is that it is not taxing to your system. You can do LISS on days you train bigger body parts like your legs or back. LISS is also my preferred cardio for contest prep athletes. For contest athletes the goal is to preserve muscle mass. With HIIT cardio you will use more glycogen compared to LISS cardio, and like I said earlier it is very taxing to your nervous system. So if muscle preservation is your goal, you can just add in more volume to your current training, and leave LISS type cardio sessions for later when reaching low body fat levels.

A sample workout schedule for using LISS/HIIT might look something like this:

Day 1: Upper Body 4x 6–8

Day 2: Lower Body 3x 10–12 (LISS)

Day 3: OFF/HIIT

Day 4: Upper Body 3x 10–12

Day 5: Lower Body 4x 6–8 (LISS)

Day 6: OFF/HIIT

Day 7: OFF/HIIT

Science of Supplements

Before I dig deep into this chapter, if I am being completely honest, this will be the *least* important chapter of the entire book. Most of you have spent, or currently spend, a lot of money on supplements. If im being honest most are a waste of money. They can only help if you are following your nutrition plan 100 percent and have a program set up for progression. With that being said, there are some supplements that can help.

Now, I feel that it is important not to just give you a list of supplements and tell you what they do. I'm also going to tell you the optimal dosage. I see far too many companies that have proprietary blends, under dosed supplements, or supplements that haven't even been shown to work in humans.

In this chapter, I'm going to list what I believe to be the most beneficial supplements and their proper dosage for building muscle and losing fat. And always make sure you are medically cleared to take anything.

There are some basic supplements I think everyone should consider buying. Not that they are magic, but I feel most people can benefit from protein powders, fiber, and multivitamins. I list these three because they can help you stay on track with macronutrients and micronutrients. I believe that most people end up undereating protein, don't eat enough fibrous foods, and thus don't get enough vitamins and minerals.

Protein Powders

I honestly believe these should be in your diet. People under consume protein all the time. Now, there are tons of different protein powders on the market. I'm not going to recommend a brand or tell you that my blend or form is better. What I am going to tell you are the kinds I think are more beneficial, practical, and cost effective. You should only take protein powders to hit your daily intake of protein.

1. **Whey Protein**
    Keeping it practical, this is probably one of the most beneficial. Whey protein powders fall into the category of fast digesting, which means they will go into your system a little faster than other forms. Whey, as I stated earlier in the Muscle Protein Synthesis section, has roughly 12 percent leucine. That would require about 30–35 grams of protein from whey to maximize leucine from a single dose and cause the greatest amount of muscle protein synthesis to occur. That's being optimal. Most whey protein powders have around 25 grams per serving. So this makes it the king when it comes to protein powders. One of the only down sides is that because it is fast digesting, you may not feel full.

2. **Casein Protein**

Casein protein falls into the category of slow digesting. Again, most protein powders have around 25 grams per serving. Casein also has a lower amount of leucine per gram compared to whey protein. Casein has roughly 8 percent leucine. So, to match leucine levels, it would take around 50 grams for the same muscle protein synthesis response as you would get from whey at 30–35 grams per serving. Now, this doesn't mean it's useless. I actually like casein because it is slow digesting and you might feel fuller for longer.

Now both whey and casein are not some magical muscle building secret. The reason I like protein powders is that I don't like eating food all the time. Generally, it's easier to drink something than it is to eat something. They are also very convenient. If you are out and about, you can drink these at anytime. The overall reason to drink something like whey or casein is to hit your total amount of protein for the day. They also usually don't have a lot of other added calories from things such as carbohydrates and fats, making them a good choice to hit total amounts of protein without searching the cabinets for something that doesn't have carbohydrates and fats. In that case, I would rather drink a shake, than have to eat something like chicken by itself!

Protein Spiking

There are some really great protein powders and some that are really bad. So, how do you choose? Learning how to read a label is important because some companies are being sued for not really listing what is in the powder. One of the biggest things to look out for is protein spiking. Spiking the level of nitrogen in a powder is a dirty trick and cheap way to throw off a test that is supposed to measure protein amounts. The current way the test is done is to measure the amount of nitrogen, which is then used to determine protein amounts. A nitrogen test is done because protein is made up of amino acids. This is accurate if they are made up of complete proteins.

Unfortunately, some companies will use extra amino acids usually found in the "other ingredients" list, such as glycine and taurine. Having added amino acids will definitely change the outcome of the nitrogen test, and the label may not be accurate.

For example, a whey protein powder might claim to have 25 grams of protein on the label. If the company added 5 grams of the amino acid glycine, you really would be only getting 20 grams of a complete protein, although the label will show 25 grams. Thus, having 5 grams of an amino acid won't have benefit for building muscle.

Another big thing is not using proteogenic type

amino acids. Proteogenics are amino acids that are used to build proteins in the body such as muscle tissue. Not every amino acid is used for muscle tissue. If that was the case, I and everyone else would look like the Incredible Hulk. There are a lot of things in the body protein is used for besides increasing muscle. One really popular amino acid I end up seeing in protein powders is taurine, used mostly because it's really cheap. So 25 grams of protein will show on the label even if there are 5 grams of taurine. You are paying for 25 grams but are only getting 20 grams.

So how can you tell if it's really protein or really just a bunch of amino acids? Well, you really can't. It may even be 5 grams of glycine and 5 grams of taurine, leaving you with only 15 grams of actual protein when you think you are getting 25 grams. So be leery if you see single amino acids in the other ingredients list.

Fiber

Fiber is one of those things I feel that people, including me, lack as well. As I said in the beginning, the recommendation for fiber intake is around 0.2 grams per pound of bodyweight. So, if you are someone who weighs 150 pounds, your fiber intake for the day is around 30 grams. If you have a hard time eating certain vegetables that contain fiber, getting fiber in the form of powders or pills can be beneficial. If you do the powder version, you can easily add this to a protein shake or any other drink.

Multitamins

If you are like most people, you probably don't eat all your vegetables. Vitamins and minerals are something people lack. On some days you might be doing well, while on others you might not do so great. On days that you work out, you can lose vitamins and minerals such as vitamin B, zinc, and copper through spending more energy on things like recovery. Getting a good multivitamin to more or less to cover your basic needs will be beneficial.

Advanced

I believe that the items in this section are not really necessary, although they can be beneficial for long term muscle growth or fat loss. If they can help you get a few more repetitions or be more focused, then they can help your long-term success.

Preworkout

There are a ton of preworkout supplements on the market. I actually take some myself but also believe a lot are under dosed, although I do think supplement companies are getting better. So, when making or buying your own, here are some I recommend being the first ones you should consider.

Creatine (3–5 grams per day)

Creatine is probably the most basic thing you should look at. I do list it in the preworkout section, but it can be taken at any time of the day and be beneficial. It just might make it more convenient to take it as part of a preworkout routine. Creatine monohydrate is probably the best bang for your buck, as it's one of the cheapest and most researched supplements on the face of the earth. It has been shown to increase muscle mass and strength and help with overall performance.

How does it work?

Adenosine tri-phosphate (ATP) is the energy source used by muscle to generate muscle contraction. ATP is basically broken down and loses a phosphate molecule, creating adenosine di-phosphate (ADP) and phosphate. The single phosphate will be reused again to form ATP. The main benefit is that it helps with taking that phosphate and creating ATP. With more ADP than ATP, energy and output will begin to slow down, yet this process is short lived. Only about five to ten seconds of this system is used as the primary energy source. Then other systems take over, such as the glycolytic pathway. There are other benefits, such as cell swelling hydration that allows you to bust out an extra rep here and there. You can see how that can be beneficial for building muscle and strength over time.

There are many different forms, but creatine

monohydrate is the most researched. Some other forms might provide benefit, but none have been shown to actually be more beneficial. So whether you get creatine monohydrate or some other form, I would still stick to the 3–5 gram dose as I recommend.

Citrulline Malate (6 grams per day)

If you have taken a preworkout supplement before, you have probably seen L-arginine. In the body, citrulline is converted over to arginine, then to nitric oxide. So why not just take arginine? Unlike citrulline, arginine actually gets broken down in the liver and intestines by the enzyme arginase. Citrulline, on the other hand, can go straight to the blood vessels. In the kidneys, citrulline is converted to arginine to be used for nitric oxide production. Research suggests that around 75 percent of L-citrulline is converted to arginine! Comparatively, arginine consumed orally that was utilized in nitric oxide production was about 1 percent. So 75 percent versus about 1 percent can make a big difference.

On the other hand, citrulline with malate attached had been shown to increase ATP production during exercise by around 35 percent. Then, after exercise, it also led to about a 20 percent increase in phosphocreatine. If you recall in the creatine section, this can work well to help with endurance and allow you to recover faster. Citrulline malate works well with creatine. This can lead to greater fatigue resistance and increased potential recovery and can increase MPS and potential muscle mass.

Betaine (2.5 grams per day)

Betaine has been shown to increase performance and increase muscle mass. I believe it should be included because it has numerous possible benefits. It has been associated with fat loss, and it has been suggested that it promotes increased creatine synthesis alongside muscle protein synthesis. So this can be beneficial by possibly allowing you to increase the amount of work being done and increase muscle protein synthesis.

Fat Loss Supplements

I actually debated on whether to talk about this or not, but I feel this is an important topic. You see them on TV with any fat loss ads, or you may walk into a gym and someone might try to sell you some kind of weight loss pill before they mention anything about training or nutrition. I know in the bodybuilding world these are treated like magic. When, in fact, most are under dosed and don't really help with fat loss.

Again, these are only an aide and can't be a substitute for training or nutrition. So before you buy something because it claims to be a "fat incinerator that shreds the pounds," there might be a reason to think twice. Don't just look at the name of the label, look at the ingredients.

There are basically three stages of fat loss and this is greatly misunderstood, not just from companies selling diet pills but in general exercise and cardio as well. You can look at them as stages, but these occur simultaneously throughout the entire day.

1. **Lipolysis (release)**

   Lipolysis is the release and reduction of stored fat from a cell. I like to picture a water balloon losing water.

2. **Transport**

   Now, just because it's released doesn't mean it will be actually used. Fat can actually go back to the cell, more or less filling the water balloon back up again. You actually have to get it to the mitochondria of the cell for it to be used as fuel.

3. **Oxidation (Burn)**

   Once you get fat to the mitochondria, it still doesn't mean it's going to be used. It can still go back and be restored. This can be prevented mostly by exercise and very minimally by supplements.

Caffeine (100–200 mg per day)

I feel caffeine is used quite a bit. It can be beneficial for a lot of different things, including concentration, strength, and fat loss, but I think people overdo it sometimes. Caffeine is helpful in the sense that it helps with lipolysis and fat burning. In relation to fat loss, a study has shown that it increased lipolysis by around 70 percent. However, what you should be looking at is how much is actually used.

That same study showed that around 30 percent was actually oxidized, so that means about 40 percent went back to storage. Now, I recommend 100–200 milligrams. An average cup of coffee contains around 150 milligrams. If you don't use caffeine products or use them that often, a low dose of 100 milligrams will be sufficient. If you drink something like coffee numerous times a day, the receptors to which caffeine binds won't bind that well. So, you can use a little higher dose of around 200 milligrams. Some people have used doses of around 300–500 milligrams. I suggest not overdoing it as caffeine has a half-life, the amount of time it stays in your system, of around six hours. So when taking caffeine err on the side of caution. If you find yourself using more and more, it would best to take a break from using it even though it can be a great potential fat burner.

Green Tea (200–500 milligrams per day)

Green tea is a great fat burner. Green tea contains compounds called catechins, with the main one being EGCG. Catechins are responsible for a thermogenic type effect, so you might feel a little bit hotter and might sweat more. EGCG inhibits an enzyme that is responsible for breaking down norepinephrine.

Norepinephrine is a neurotransmitter that is involved in the regulation of your metabolism and also aids in fat burning. Thus, this will help with elevation of norepinephrine and encourage fat burning. I would suggest taking a lower dose first, as some people might get an upset stomach.

L-Carnitine (1–2 grams per day)

L-Carnitine will help with the transportation of fatty acids to the mitochondria. Once they pass into the mitochondria, they can be oxidized and are ready to create ATP. Carnitine also has some other benefits such as in muscle tissue to increase the androgen receptor density. So, it may help promote the formation of muscle tissue. You can take this before a workout, after a workout, or in the morning.

Review

Although supplements are not necessary, some can be really beneficial. Whether it is for something basic such as a protein powder to hit an overall protein total for the day, something to give you that extra energy that will allow you to do a few more repetitions, or something that will aid in fat loss, these are the ones I recommend and find most beneficial.

Sustainable Diet

At the very beginning of this book, I said that this will be different than your typical diet. This book won't tell you what to eat. In order to be sustainable, your diet should be composed of foods you actually enjoy eating, right? It's not going to be bland chicken, broccoli, and rice eating from Tupperware, unless you actually like to eat that kind of food. The truth is, you don't have to eat the same thing every day. If you made it this far and I didn't bore you, that's great!

I hope you did not just jump right to this section. Throughout the book, I actually wanted you to learn, and know the reasons behind this entire chapter. The rest of this section is about building something you can use. By this point you should have starting calories and starting macronutrients and have an understanding of metabolic adaptations, practical applications, and some basic supplements. Whether you are a stay-at-home parent, someone with a busy work schedule where you have to eat out more often then you should, or a competitive bodybuilding athlete, this section is the accumulation of the entire book.

Up until now, this entire book has been about understanding flexible dieting. You have probably worked with a trainer, nutritionist, or prep coach before, and they might have had a "this is the best approach" mentality. Or you have may have heard of keto, carb cycling, or low-carb high-fat (LCHF) diets.

I like to think of all these ways to diet as tools in

a toolbox. They each serve their individual purpose, and some tools might work better in different points in time. I'm not going to say this is the best way to diet, I will use other types of dieting when necessary with different people, but the entire purpose of this book was to allow for something sustainable and something that allows you to keep fat off after your diet, whether that was to just lose ten pounds and fit into a dress or whether you are a competitive body builder.

Carb Cycling

Carb cycling isn't a new term. It actually is used a lot by diet coaches. For one, it allows you to, well, eat carbs! There might be some science behind it, as it might have an impact on the mitochondria. The mitochondria are the powerhouse of the cell, and site of energy production. Having low days, it might suggest an increase in mitochondria. Thus, it might have an impact on fat oxidation.

As you know, fat loss isn't linear, meaning it's not a straight line. Carb cycling is exactly what it sounds like, cycling of carbohydrates. In short, it's alternating between low, medium, and high carbohydrate days, or variations of those. This can either be by days, or even by weeks. I like to view it as stair steps. There are many different ways of carb cycling, but I'm just going to show you two.

Refeed days are optimal in that you are accounting for everything, and if you are doing a flexible dieting style of dieting, then you are not cheating on your diet.

Example maintenance calories: 2,205 calories (150 grams protein, 45 grams fat, and 300 grams carbohydrate)

Carb Cycle example #1: slight deficit, followed by two smaller refeed days.

Day 1:   150 g protein, 45 g fat, 300 g carbs (high day/refeed day)

Day 2:   150 g protein, 45 g fat, 200 g carbs (medium day)

Day 3:   150 g protein, 45 g fat, 200 g carbs (medium day)

Day 4:   150 g protein, 45 g fat, 155 g carbs (low day/off day)

Day 5:   150 g protein, 45 g fat, 300 g carbs (high day/refeed day)

Day 6:   150 g protein, 45 g fat, 200 g carbs (medium day)

Day 7:   150 g protein, 45 g fat, 200 g carbs (medium day)

Carb Cycle example #2: slight deficit, followed by one bigger refeed days.

Day 1:   150 g protein, 45 g fat, 200 g carbs (medium day)

Day 2:   150 g protein, 45 g fat, 200 g carbs (medium day)

Day 3:   150 g protein, 45 g fat, 200 g carbs (medium day)

Day 4:   150 g protein, 45 g fat, 155 g

carbs (low day/off day)

Day 5:   150 g protein, 45 g fat, 200 g
          carbs (medium day)

Day 6:   150 g protein, 45 g fat, 200 g
          carbs (medium day)

Day 7:   150 g protein, 45 g fat, 450 g
          carbs (high day/refeed day)

I favor carb cycling mostly because by following a diet that is really restrictive on carbohydrates, especially at the beginning or for the entire duration of the diet, it can slow metabolic rate, decrease leptin levels, and possibly cause you to lose strength. So which example is more optimal? I think that really depends on how difficult it is for you to lose body fat. Neither has been shown to more beneficial compared to the other.

Some people might be able to use both, while others might benefit from just doing one. For one, leptin is not magical as I said earlier. It is only responsible for around a 7 percent increase in metabolic rate. I will use both versions at various points throughout dieting. But, ultimately, it comes down to something you can follow, so I'm going to use #1 as the example for the rest of the chapter.

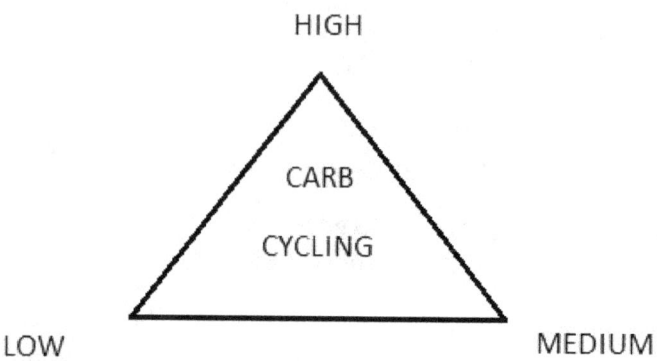

HIGH

CARB

CYCLING

LOW   MEDIUM

Setting Up Your Carb Cycle

Maintenance calories are what I had you figure out at the beginning of this book. Maintenance calories are what your body is used to consuming so that you are neither losing weight nor gaining weight.

So using this example again, you may come up with the following plan:

Example maintenance calories: 2,205 calories (150 grams protein, 45 grams fat, and 300 grams carbohydrates)

Carb Cycle example #1: slight deficit, followed by two smaller refeed days.

Day 1:   150 g protein, 45 g fat, 300 g
          carbs (high day/refeed day)

Day 2:   150 g protein, 45 g fat, 200 g

carbs (medium day)

Day 3:   150 g protein, 45 g fat, 200 g
           carbs (medium day)

Day 4:   150 g protein, 45 g fat, 155 g
           carbs (low day/off day)

Day 5:   150 g protein, 45 g fat, 300 g
           carbs (high day/refeed day)

Day 6:   150 g protein, 45 g fat, 200 g
           carbs (medium day)

Day 7:   150 g protein, 45 g fat, 200 g
           carbs (medium day)

To figuring out your high day/refeed day, we will just be using your maintenance calories. Throughout adjusting your carbohydrate intake, protein, and fat, totals will remain the same. Now these starting numbers are not set in stone. It depends on the rate of loss that was covered earlier. For some, this might be too fast, while for others it might be too slow, but this will be a good starting point.

Start with the medium day calories: (1,805 calories: 150 grams protein, 45 grams fat, and 200 grams carbohydrates). Take 20 percent of this total (0.2 multiplied by total maintenance calories).

So in this example, 0.2 x 2205 = 441 calories. Now take that and divide by 4 (the amount of calories in 1 gram of carbohydrates. Yes, I know, math!). You should come up with a number around 110. This will be the amount you will take off from your maintenance carbohydrates. I rounded to 200.

Now, use the low/off day calories (1,625 calories: 150 grams protein, 45 grams fat, and 155 grams carbohydrates). Take 10 percent (0.1 multiplied by total medium day calories).

In this example, 0.1 x 1,805 = 180.5 calories. Now take that and divide by 4. You will come up with a number around 45. Now, these are not some magical secret percentages, nor do I claim them to be, a lot of people might follow something similar to this. This will just be an initial deficit, a slightly lower amount of calories than what you are maintaining at.

Making Adjustments

There are two ways to make adjustments, and that is by either increasing energy expenditure or by decreasing calorie intake. In this section I will break up non-competitors and competitors. As I said earlier, cardio, whether HIIT or LISS, is just for assistance when needed. I am not fond of changing this first, but I recommend starting with two HIIT sessions two times per week. If you can't do a HIIT session, I would start off with doing fifteen minutes of LISS. If you are a competitor I would start off with only doing two LISS sessions. If you recall in the HIIT/LISS chapter, if you start off doing something like six days a week and stall, there really isn't much you can do besides keep dropping calories. So start off with doing two sessions a week. Some of you may not need to adjust from here. This all depends on how much you have to lose. This will also determine how long you should be dieting and how fast you should be losing fat. If you are someone who has more than twenty pounds to lose, you can be safe and lose around two to three pounds a week, making around twenty or more weeks of dieting. Then, if you are someone who has, let's say, twelve pounds or less, go off of the ROL rate of loss of one to two pounds a week, putting you roughly at one week per pound of dieting.

If you are someone who needs to make adjustments, the only thing in the diet you will be changing is the medium days and low days. Keep the refeed days the same. This will only be if you don't see results in the first three to four weeks. In some cases, if you haven't been working out, you may actually build some initial muscle. This won't happen throughout the entire course of dieting, but can at the beginning. So instead of looking at the scale, get a body fat test done. You don't have to spend a lot; a simple caliper test will do. I would get a body fat check done about every month and have a notebook to record body fat measurements. Second, take pictures and measurements. When dieting for myself I wake up and take a picture about once a week, in the same position, in front of the same mirror. The weight might be the same on the scale, but if you take pictures and measurements, you can actually see and measure progress.

Yes, I just said don't rely on the scale, but upon waking up in the morning and without drinking water or eating, get on a scale if you have one. This will be the most accurate way to track scale progress. Okay, back to making changes to medium and low days. If you don't see any progress after three to four weeks, then we can adjust nutrition and cardio.

For medium and low days, we are only going to adjust by about 5 percent. So you will take your total calories on medium days and multiply that by 5 percent. Using the same example, that gives you about 90 calories. Then divide by four and get roughly 20 grams of carbohydrates to take away from your medium days. You will do the same exact thing for your low day, using 5 percent of low day's calories.

You should come up with these numbers.

OLD MEDIUM DAY (1,805 calories): 150 grams protein, 45 grams fat, 200 grams carbohydrates

OLD LOW/OFF DAY (1,625 calories): 150 grams protein, 45 grams fat, 155 grams carbohydrates

NEW MEDIUM DAY (1,725 calories): 150 grams protein, 45g fat, 180 grams carbohydrates

NEW LOW/OFF DAY (1,525 calories): 150 grams protein, 45 grams fat, 130 grams carbohydrates

After making nutrition adjustments, now let's adjust cardio. If you have initially been doing two sessions of HIIT two times a week, change the number of intervals from two to three, and add in an additional day of HIIT increasing from two days to three days per week.

If you are doing LISS two days a week for fifteen minutes, add two to three days and increase time from fifteen minutes to twenty minutes. Now allow at least one week for adjustments.

Recall that fat loss isn't linear. Some people might

have a hard time losing weight, while others won't have to adjust much or add in a ton of cardio. If you go another three to four weeks, and you are being consistent, you can adjust again exactly like before around the eight-week mark. Eight-weeks is just a guideline, if you want to be more precise, go off of ROL, and adjust to stay at a rate of one to two pounds per week. You can keep adding additional HIIT sessions up to seven intervals, although I wouldn't recommend doing more than five days per week. You can do six, but you also risk taking a toll on your strength, including possible muscle loss. If you are a competitor I would recommend adding in a little more volume to your training instead of HIIT, and stick with LISS closer to your competition. If doing LISS, I recommend not doing any more than five days per week and for no longer than thirty minutes. Again you really risk losing strength and muscle. If you can adjust nutrition first before adding in more days or sessions of cardio, that would be more optimal. Personally I will go as long as I can without doing cardio, and only use it when I feel that I need too.

If you go back to the HIIT/LISS chapter, you can also make adjustments using a combination.

Here is a sample seven-day plan:

Day 1: HIIT

Day 2: LISS

Day 3: HIIT

Day 4: LISS

Day 5: HIIT

Day 6: OFF

Day 7: OFF

A Word of Advice

Life isn't perfect, and neither is dieting. It's not going to be an easy straight line. There will be days when you fall off, but it's never about being perfect. Even I am not perfect. Now, I am not saying it's okay to go out and have a free week of eating. If you lose track, life happens, and you eat a little over or under, don't feel guilty. I do the same thing. The only thing I ask of you is to be consistent.

Reaching a goal isn't about being perfect all the time. It's not a simple path. If it was, I'm pretty sure the new "insert detox tea name here" would be prescribed to everyone to take! Reaching a goal is about consistency over time. It's about battling through your setbacks to come back stronger. Lastly, be real with yourself. If you find yourself not being as consistent in the gym as much as you would like, or maybe you find yourself enjoying a little more food once in a while, be real. Reflect on the reasons why you are not being consistent with working out and figure out why you are not being as consistent with nutrition.

If you can figure out the reasons why, then you can always power through them. If you find yourself eating less because of lack of time, then you might have to wake up earlier in the day to prepare foods. I struggled with this as a student going to 7:30 a.m classes. But whatever you end up doing, don't beat yourself up for it. I see a lot of people get frustrated and try to overcompensate by doing a ton of cardio the next day or by barely eating anything. Don't do it! One day isn't going to hurt. Just get your mind-set back on track and get prepared for the next day.

1. Stick to your diet.
2. Make changes if fat loss stalls.
3. Be real with yourself.
4. Be happy with progress, even if it's slow.
5. Go ahead and eat that donut (just track it)!

Keep going until you get where you want to be. Then get ready for reverse dieting.

Reverse Dieting

Reverse dieting is a big topic. Reverse dieting is the process that you follow after a prolonged period of dieting, where you increase calories over time. Just like dieting down to lose body fat, this is also a systematic approach to increase calories over time. There is no need to stay in a deficit, like a lot of clean-eating diets. They generally give you a diet to follow for twelve weeks. You diet for twelve weeks, but then what? Or maybe you just got done with a bodybuilding show. What do you do next?

The overall idea of reverse dieting is to

1. avoid a lot of excess body fat regain beyond what you are comfortable with;
2. increase overall metabolic rate;
3. allow for hormones levels to increase;
4. get back to training harder/restore lost muscle; and
5. get back to a normal psychological point.

If you go back to the metabolic adaptation chapter, your metabolism changes over time. There is actually no such thing as a damaged metabolism. With prolonged dieting, you generally get a decreased overall TDEE.

For example, after a bodybuilding contest some people blow up. After the show is over, they hit up every food joint within sight and eat everything within arm's reach. I have seen it a lot. There really isn't a problem with this for one day. It's the prolonged days of binge eating that lead to serious problems. With a metabolism that is low, you are basically used to your dieting calories. So once you go off your diet and eat two to three times as much as you normally would for multiple days, this will result in a lot of postdiet fat regain. Yes, I said fat. A lot of people mistake this for muscle growth, but just because you put pack on weight doesn't mean it's all coming in the form of muscle tissue, especially if you go right back into a caloric surplus.

Using the example before, let's assume example maintenance is 2,205 calories (150 grams protein, 45 grams fat, and 300 grams carbohydrates).

This is your old maintenance calories. With overall metabolism being lower and loss of muscle mass if you are a competitor, you won't be jumping right back to these calories. Your old maintenance would be a surplus and lead to possible fat gain by not just filling out old cells, but also by creating new fat cells.

With application, there will be a difference in how you should approach this, whether you are a competitor or not. If you are a competitor there is no need to be stage lean all the time. This is where a lot of reverse dieting is done wrong in that some coaches think it's literally just doing the opposite to add calories back in. I don't see the need to be in a deficit for twelve to twenty weeks. For a competitor you would be wasting a lot of potential offseason time.

Right away, it will be okay to bring up calories quickly initially. However, I'm not going to say, "Oh, okay, let's just eat until I get to a new maintenance." Like most competitors, you are probably fantasizing about the next thing you can stuff your face with (I know I usually am). The chance of overshooting is greater. Mentally, dieting is hard, especially for competition. So, I also believe the psychological point of reverse dieting is just as important, but you should do it systematically with set calories and macronutrients.

On the other had if you don't compete and just dieted for general fat loss, I would normally recommend a slower revere diet.

Okay, so let's say just got done with a diet, and your current nutrient intake is 1,245 calories (150 grams protein, 45 grams fats, 60 grams carbohydrates).

From this point on, it's about monitoring since we don't know your new maintenance, and it's about going slow. Take pictures, measurements, and even get a body fat test done. From here on out, only add about ten carbohydrates per week and pull back cardio slowly to where gradually you are only doing two days per week or none at all. If you get to a point where you are not gaining weight, this is your new maintenance. From here, you can decide where you want to go, whether that's to stay where you are or go into a caloric surplus to build muscle.

For more of a post-competition-day set-up (assuming contest conditioning), let's assume you are at 1,245 calories (150 grams protein, 45 grams fats, 60 grams carbohydrates).

That Saturday night go out with the family, enjoy a meal. Then on that initial postshow Sunday, be conscious of how much you eat, preferring to hit a minimum protein and a minimum fat amount and being cautious of carbohydrates roughly hitting about three to four meals that are portioned out. Following that coming Monday, take about 20 percent of total calories (1,245), divide by four, and add to your carbohydrates. You should now have roughly 1,485 calories (150 grams protein, 45 grams fats, 120 grams carbohydrates)

This should put you really close to new maintenance calories. Once you get to maintenance, stay here for about two weeks duration.

From here on out it, will be the same thing. If you are female, only add back about ten carbohydrates a week. If you are male, add in about twenty carbohydrates a week and gradually pull back cardio until you are only doing two days per week or none at all.

The overall goal is to get back to feeling normal, back to the point where you are at a healthy mind-set viewing food and not wanting to dive into the fridge to see how much you can fit in your mouth. You ultimately want to get back to a normal range of hormone function. Once the reverse dieting is done, you may get going on your off season to create new muscle and increase calories. This will allow for a good starting point for dieting for your next competition, or allow you to maintain your current body weight.

Reverse dieting isn't some magical new dieting trick, but it can be a useful tool to keep hard earned progress. I hope you have some new insight into reverse dieting and its importance in getting you back to feeling normal.

The whole point of this entire book was to create something you can do for life. It's not a quick fix diet.

Although I do not guarantee results for everyone, some of you will get great results, while others might have to battle each and every day. It will all come back to consistency, determination, and the willpower to work toward your own personal end goal. You now should have a great understanding of calories, macronutrients, micronutrients, metabolic adaptations, setting up a diet, and how to stay leaner and get back to feeling normal through reverse dieting. To everyone reading, I hope you find value in this book, and thank you for letting me be a part of your own journey.

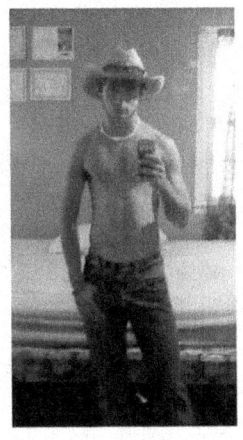 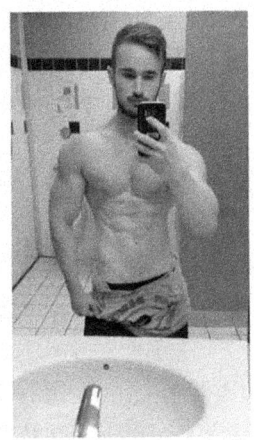

I'm being real with everyone! On the left, this was me at about 133 pounds. On the right, I was about 155 pounds. Granted, I don't look like this all the time. This was right after a workout. As you can probably see, I had below average genetics, but what I did have was determination. I'm not expecting you to be perfect. It's about getting started, being consistent, and continually learning.

REFERENCES

Antonio, J., et al. The effects of a high protein diet on indices of health and body composition – a crossover trial in resistance-trained men. Int Soc Sports Nutr 13:3, 2016.

Bailey SJ, Blackwell JR, Lord T, Vanhatalo A, Winyard PG, Jones AM. l-Citrulline supplementation improves O2 uptake kinetics and high-intensity exercise performance in humans. J ApplPhysiol (1985). 2015 Aug 15;119(4):385-95

Bowman MP, *et al* Effect of dietary fat and cholesterol on plasma lipids and lipoprotein fractions in normolipidemic men . *J Nutr.* (1988)

Branch JD. Effect of creatine supplementation and performance: a meta-analysis. Int J Sport NutrExercMetab. 2003

Candow DG, Vogt E, Johannsmeyer S, Forbes SC, Farthing JP.
Strategic creatine supplementation and resistance training in healthy older adults.
ApplPhysiolNutrMetab. 2015 Jul;40(7):689-94.

Cholewa JM1, Guimarães-Ferreira L, Zanchi NE. Amino Acids. Effects of betaine on performance and body composition: a review of recent findings and potential mechanisms. 2014 Aug;46(8):1785-93.

Cholewa, J. M., et al. Effects of betaine on body composition, performance, and homocysteine thiolactone. Journal of The International Society of Sports Nutrition 10:39, 2013.

Dirlewanger M, di Vetta V, Guenat E, Battilana P, Seematter G, Schneiter P, Jequier E, Tappy L: Effects of short-term carbohydrate or fat overfeeding on energy expenditure and plasma leptin concentrations in healthy female subjects. Int J Obes Relat Metab Disord. 2000, 24: 1413-1418. 10.1038/sj.ijo.0801395.

Doucet E, St-Pierre S, Almeras N, Despres JP, Bouchard C, Tremblay A: Evidence for the existence of adaptive thermogenesis during weight loss. Br J Nutr. 2001, 85: 715-723. 10.1079/BJN2001348.

Francaux M1, Demeure R, Goudemant JF, Poortmans JR. Effect of exogenous creatine supplementation on muscle PCr metabolism. Int J Sports Med. 2000 Feb;21(2):139-45.

Katan MB, *et al* <u>Saturated fat and heart disease</u> . *Am J Clin Nutr.* (2010)

Le Plénier S, Walrand S, Noirt R, Cynober L, Moinard C. Effects of leucine and citrulline versus non-essential amino acids on muscle protein synthesis in fasted rat: a common activation pathway? Amino Acids. 2012 Sep;43(3):1171-8.

Levine JA: Non-exercise activity thermogenesis (NEAT). Best Pract Res Clin Endocrinol Metab. 2002, 16: 679-702. 10.1053/beem.2002.0227.

Longland, T. M., et al. Higher compared with lower dietary protein during an energy deficit combined with intense exercise promotes greater lean mass gain and fat mass loss: a randomized trial. The American Journal of Clinical Nutrition, in press, 2016.

Maestu J, Jurimae J, Valter I, Jurimae T: Increases in ghrelin and decreases in leptin without altering adiponectin during extreme weight loss in male competitive bodybuilders. Metabolism. 2008, 57: 221-225. 10.1016/j.metabol.2007.09.004.

Margetic S, Gazzola C, Pegg GG, Hill RA: Leptin: a review of its peripheral actions and interactions. Int J Obes Relat Metab Disord. 2002, 26: 1407-1433. 10.1038/sj.ijo.0802142.

Miles CW, Wong NP, Rumpler WV, Conway J: Effect of circadian variation in energy expenditure, within-subject variation and weight reduction on thermic effect of food. Eur J Clin Nutr. 1993, 47: 274-284.

Moinard C, Le Plenier S, Noirez P, Morio B, Bonnefont-Rousselot D, Kharchi C, Ferry A, Neveux N, Cynober L, Raynaud-Simon A. Citrulline Supplementation Induces Changes in Body Composition and Limits Age-Related Metabolic Changes in Healthy Male Rats. J Nutr. 2015 Jul;145(7):1429-37

Mozaffarian D, Micha R, Wallace S Effects on coronary heart disease of increasing polyunsaturated fat in place of saturated fat: a systematic review and meta-analysis of randomized controlled trials . PLoS Med. (2010)

Nagaya N, Uematsu M, Oya H, Sato N, Sakamaki F, Kyotani S, Ueno K, Nakanishi N, Yamagishi M, Miyatake K. Short-term oral administration of L-arginine improves hemodynamics and exercise capacity in patients with precapillary pulmonary hypertension. Am J RespirCrit Care Med. 2001 Mar;163(4):887-91.

Norton, Layne E et al. "Leucine Content of Dietary Proteins Is a Determinant of Postprandial Skeletal Muscle Protein Synthesis in Adult Rats." *Nutrition & Metabolism* 9 (2012): 67. *PMC*. Web. 20 Oct. 2016.

Osowska S, Duchemann T, Walrand S, Paillard A, Boirie Y, Cynober L, Moinard C. Citrulline modulates muscle protein metabolism in old malnourished rats. Am J PhysiolEndocrinolMetab. 2006 Sep;291(3):E582-6.

Osowska S, Moinard C, Neveux N, Loï C, and Cynober L. Citrulline increases arginine pools and restores nitrogen balance after massive intestinal resection. Gut 53: 1781–1786, 2004.

Pérez-Guisado J, Jakeman PM. Citrulline malate enhances athletic anaerobic performance and relieves muscle soreness. J Strength Cond Res. 2010 May;24(5):1215-22.

Raatz,SK: Reduced glycemic index and glycemic load diets do not increase the effects of energy restriction on weight loss and insulin sensitivity in obese men and women. J.Nutr 2005 Oct;135(10):2387-91.

Ravussin E, Burnand B, Schutz Y, Jequier E: Energy expenditure before and during energy restriction in obese patients. Am J Clin Nutr. 1985, 41: 753-759.

Rossow LM, Fukuda DH, Fahs CA, Loenneke JP, Stout JR: Natural bodybuilding competition preparation and recovery: a 12-month case study. Int J Sports Physiol Perform. 2013, 8: 582-592.

Rosenbaum M, Leibel RL: Adaptive thermogenesis in humans. Int J Obes. 2010, 34 (Suppl 1): S47-S55.

Siri-Tarino PW, *et al* Meta-analysis of prospective cohort studies evaluating the association of saturated fat with cardiovascular disease . *Am J Clin Nutr*. (2010)

Solomonson, L. P., et al. The caveolar nitric oxide synthase/arginine regeneration system for NO production in endothelial cells. J ExpBiol 206:2083–2087, 2003.

Stone MH1, Sanborn K, Smith LL, O'Bryant HS, Hoke T, Utter AC, Johnson RL, Boros R, Hruby J, Pierce KC, Stone ME, Garner B. Effects of in-season (5 weeks) creatine and pyruvate supplementation on anaerobic performance and bodycomposition in American football players. Int J Sport Nutr. 1999 Jun;9(2):146-65.

Ventura G, Noirez P, Breuillé D, Godin JP, Pinaud S, Cleroux M, Choisy C, Le Plénier S, Bastic V, Neveux N, Cynober L, Moinard C. Effect of citrulline on muscle functions during moderate dietary restriction in healthy adult rats. Amino Acids. 2013 Nov;45(5):1123-31.

Volek, J.S., et al. Effects of a high-fat diet on postabsorptive and postprandial testosterone responses to a fat-rich meal. Metabolism 50(11): 1,351-1,355, 2001.

Volek, J.S., et al. Testosterone and cortisol in relationship to dietary nutrients and resistance exercise. Journal of Applied Physiology 82(1): 49-54, 1997.

Walberg JL, Leidy MK, Sturgill DJ, Hinkle DE, Ritchey SJ, Sebolt DR. "Macronutrient content of a hypoenergy diet affects nitrogen retention and muscle function in weight lifters." Int J Sports Med. 1988 Aug; 9(4):261-6.

Wang Q, *et al* Effect of omega-3 fatty acids supplementation on endothelial function: A meta-analysis of randomized controlled trials . *Atherosclerosis*. (2012)

Weigle DS: Contribution of decreased body mass to diminished thermic effect of exercise in reduced-obese men. Int J Obes. 1988, 12: 567-578.

Woodside JV, McKinley MC, Young IS <u>Saturated and trans fatty acids and coronary heart disease</u> . *Curr Atheroscler Rep.* (2008)

Zinchenko, A., & Henselmans, M. (2016). Metabolic Damage: do Negative Metabolic Adaptations During Underfeeding Persist After Refeeding in Non-Obese Populations? *Medical Research Archives, 4*(8). doi:10.18103/mra.v4i8.908

ABOUT THE AUTHOR

Keegan Brown received his bachelors of science in fitness and wellness with a minor in biology from Park University. Keegan is a certified personal trainer, nutritionist, author, physique coach, and owner at keeganbrown.net He has dedicated his life to the science of fitness. Fitness is his passion. He believes in using what is proven in research to dictate real-world application. Keegan has worked with people from all walks of life. For clients such as stay-at-home moms and competitive athletes, Keegan has helped people get in the best shape of their lives, all without sacrificing health. As a competitive athlete, he has won numerous awards over the course of his career. He is always striving to further his own knowledge when it comes to nutrition, health, and fitness, not just for himself but for others as well.

www.ingramcontent.com/pod-product-compliance
Lightning Source LLC
Chambersburg PA
CBHW072104280526
45788CB00006B/2388

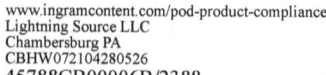